MW01293851

# 50 Protein Bars for the Special Diet

## Gluten Free, Keto, Plant Based, and Much More

BY

Julia Chiles

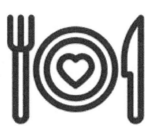

Copyright 2019 - Julia Chiles

OOOOOOOOOOOOOOOOOOOOOOOOOOOOOOOOOOOOOOOOO

# License Notes

No part of this Book can be reproduced in any form or by any means including print, electronic, scanning or photocopying unless prior permission is granted by the author.

All ideas, suggestions and guidelines mentioned here are written for informative purposes. While the author has taken every possible step to ensure accuracy, all readers are advised to follow information at their own risk. The author cannot be held responsible for personal and/or commercial damages in case of misinterpreting and misunderstanding any part of this Book

OOOOOOOOOOOOOOOOOOOOOOOOOOOOOOOOOOOOOOO

# Thanks for Purchasing My Book! - Here's Your Reward!

Thank you so much for purchasing my book! As a reward for your purchase, you can now receive free books sent to you every week. All you have to do is just subscribe to the list by entering your email address in the box below and I will send you a notification every time I have a free promotion running. The books will absolutely be free with no work at all from you! Who doesn't want free books? No one! *There are free and discounted books every day*, and an email is sent to you 1-2 days beforehand to remind you so you don't miss out. It's that easy! Enter your email now to get started!

∽ **Sign up now & get your free e-book** ∽

FIRST NAME:

YOUR EMAIL:

Refreshing *recepies*

**SIGN UP**

http://julia-chiles.subscribemenow.com

OOOOOOOOOOOOOOOOOOOOOOOOOOOOOOOOOOOO

# Table of Contents

# Introduction

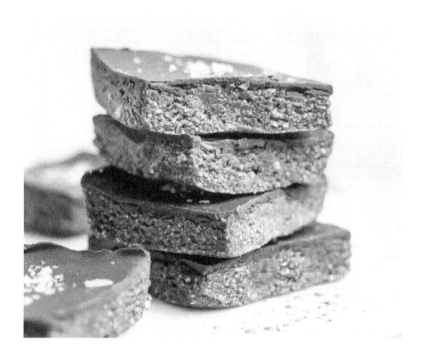

Make perfect protein bars for your active, healthy lifestyle. 50 Protein Bars for the Special Diet: Gluten Free, Keto, Plant Based, Etc. will guide you through every step! It's the perfect cookbook for those who are committed to creating quality days for themselves and their families.

# No-Bake Gluten Free Protein Bars

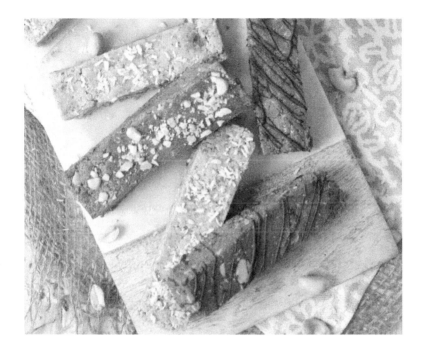

Sub honey or agave for the maple syrup!

**Makes:** 10 bars.

**Ingredients:**

- 2 1/3 cups old-fashioned certified gluten free rolled oats
- 2 tbsp gluten free protein powder -or- collagen powder
- 8-10 pitted soft Medjool dates
- 2 ½ - 3 tbsp maple syrup
- ½ teaspoon vanilla extract
- ¼ teaspoon kosher salt, optional
- 2 tbsp milk, any kind (use more if needed ½ tsp at a time
- 3 ounces unsweetened chocolate, chopped for melting
- 8 ounces bittersweet chocolate, chopped for melting

**Directions:**

Pulse oats until powder.

Add protein powder, dates, syrup, vanilla, salt, milk, and pulse 20-30 seconds or until 'tacky but not sticky".

Melt unsweetened chocolate in a microwave safe dish 10 seconds at a time, stirring after each time.

Pour melted chocolate into mixture then pour into a 9x9 pan.

Cover and refrigerate 30 minutes.

Cut into bars and dip into melted bittersweet chocolate.

# Butternut No-Bake Gluten Free Bars

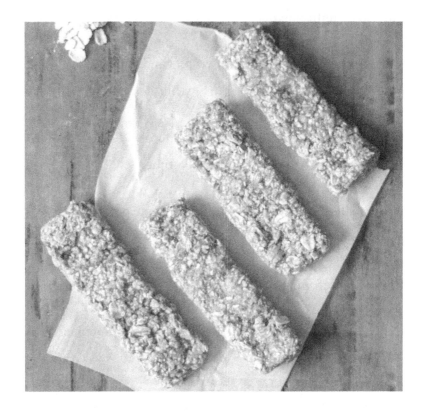

Natural peanut butter works too!

**Makes:** 8-10 bars.

**Ingredients:**

- 2 cups old-fashioned certified gluten free rolled oats
- 2 tbsp gluten free protein powder
- ¼ cup + 2 tbsp unsweetened cocoa powder (natural or Dutch-processed)
- ½ cup nut butter -or- almond butter
- 1 ½ tbsp maple syrup
- 2 tbsp milk any kind, (use more as necessary 1/3 tsp at a time)
- 3 ounces unsweetened chocolate, melted
- 8 ounces bittersweet chocolate, melted

**Directions:**

Pulse oats until powder.

Add protein powder, dates, syrup, vanilla, salt, milk, and pulse 20-30 seconds or until 'tacky but not sticky".

Melt unsweetened chocolate in a microwave safe dish 10 seconds at a time, stirring after each time.

Pour melted chocolate into mixture then pour into a 9x9 pan.

Cover and refrigerate 30 minutes.

Cut into bars and dip into melted bittersweet chocolate.

# Sweeten with Stevia Gluten Free Protein Bar

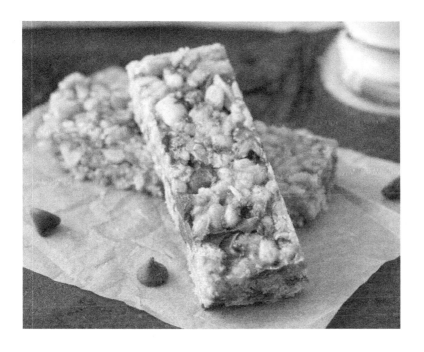

18-20 grams of protein!

**Makes:** 12-14 bars.

**Ingredients:**

- 2/3 cup of Natural Roasted Peanut Butter
- ¾ cup + 2 tsp Peanut Flour
- 1 ¼ cup Unsweetened Vanilla Almond Milk (more as need ½ tsp at a time)
- 1 ¼ cup + 1 tbsp Vanilla Brown Rice Protein Powder
- 3 oz Bittersweet Chocolate
- 35-40 Pretzel Rods gluten free
- 1 tsp of Vanilla Crème-Flavored Stevia Extract

**Directions:**

Crush pretzels and melt chocolate then combine and press into the bottom of a 9x9 pan. Keep in refrigerator until needed.

In separate bowl combine rice protein powder and peanut flour.

In pot over medium heat combine peanut butter, milk, and stevia extract.

Stir until smooth.

Let cool 1 minute and pour on top of chocolate/pretzel mixture in pan.

Distribute evenly and refrigerate covered 30 minutes -1 hour.

# Gluten Free & Vegan Friendly

# Blueberry Bars

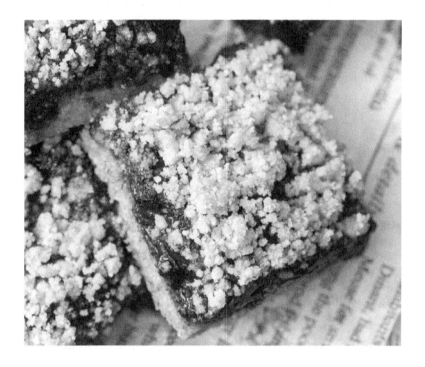

Substitute dried cranberries for the blueberries!

**Makes:** 12-14 bars.

**Ingredients:**

- 1 cup Gluten Free oats
- ½ cup whole almonds
- ½ cup dried blueberries
- 1/3 cup pistachios
- ⅓ cup ground flaxseed -or- hempseed
- ⅓ cup walnuts
- ¼ cup pepitas
- 1/5 cup sunflower seeds
- 3 ½ tbsp maple syrup or honey
- 3 ½ tbsp apple sauce
- ¾ cup almond butter

**Directions:**

In a large bowl combine oats, almonds, blueberries, pistachios, flaxseed or hempseed, walnuts, pepitas, sunflower seeds.

Add syrup or honey, applesauce, almond butter.

Mix and pour into 8x8 or 9x9 pan.

Refrigerate 45 minutes-1 hour.

Keep refrigerated or make ahead and freeze.

# Peanut Butter Protein Bars

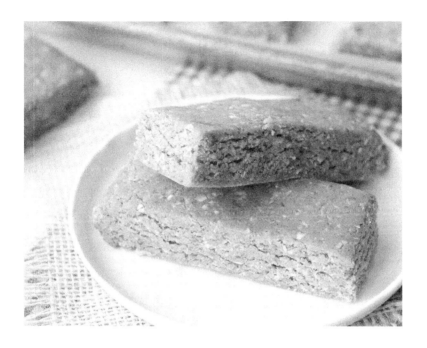

Crisped rice works in lieu of soy crisps!

**Makes:** 10-12.

## Ingredients:

- 4 ¾ cup soy crisps
- ¼ cup + 2 tbsp powdered peanut butter
- 6 tbsp (2 oz) soy protein powder
- 6 tbsp agave
- ½ c water
- ¼ cup pretzels, crushed
- 2 tbsp peanuts, crushed
- ¼ cup peanut butter chips

## Directions:

Pour 2 ½ cups of soy crisps into blender, pulse 4 times.

In pot combine soy crisps, powdered peanut butter, water, agave stir over medium-high heat.

Melt and let boil 20-30 seconds.

Pour into a pan and press down evenly.

Top with peanuts, pretzels, and chips then store in refrigerator.

# Tom's German Choco Protein Bars

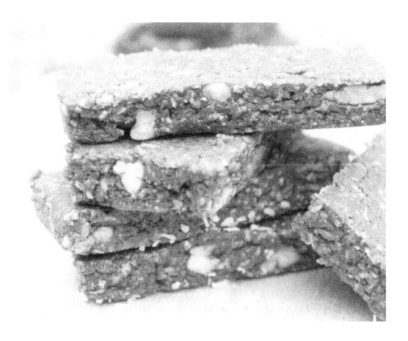

Sub walnuts or almonds for the pecans! 9 grams of protein.

**Makes:** 10-12 bars.

## Ingredients:

- ¾ cup oats
- 1/3 cup +3 ½ tbsp soy protein powder
- 4 tbsp cocoa powder
- ½ cup dates pitted, washed, and drained
- ¾ cup pecans
- 1 cup shredded coconut
- 6 tbsp brown rice syrup
- 1 tsp vanilla extract

## Directions:

Combine in a food processor oat, protein powder, and cocoa powder and grind into a powder.

Add dates, pecans, coconut, vanilla blending and adding water by the tsp until a dough forms.

Transfer to bowl and stir in chips.

Press evenly into an 8x8 or 9x9 pan, cover, and refrigerate 1 ½ hours.

# Renee's Germen Chocolate & Dried Cranberries Protein Bars

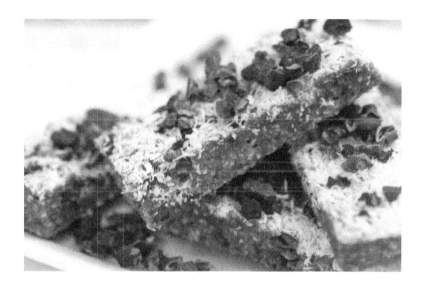

Try subbing the dried cranberries for prunes!

**Makes:** 8 – 10 bars, 9 grams of protein.

## Ingredients:

- 1 cup oats
- 8-10 scoops vegan protein powder (if scoops are 2 tbsp)
- 3 ½ tbsp cocoa powder
- 1 cup Medjool dates pitted, soak for 30 minutes
- 2/3 cup coarsely crushed pecans, divided
- 2/3 cup shredded coconut, divided
- 1/3 cup dried cranberries
- ¾ tsp vanilla extract
- ¼ tsp salt
- water as needed
- 2 ½ tbsp cacao or chocolate chips

**Directions:**

Combine in a food processor oat, protein powder, and cocoa powder and grind into a powder.

Add dates, pecans, coconut, dried cranberries, vanilla blending and adding water by the tsp until a dough form.

Transfer to bowl and stir in chips.

Press evenly into an 8x8 or 9x9 pan, cover, and refrigerate 2 hours.

# Ginger Crunch Protein Bars

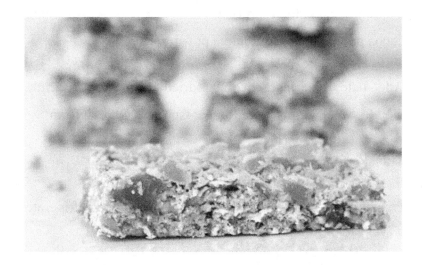

Sub turmeric for the ginger!

**Makes:** 10 bars.

**Ingredients:**

- ¾ cup + 1 tbsp. Gluten Free Old-Fashioned Rolled Oats
- ½ cup corn flakes cereal, crushed
- 3 ½ tbsp. almonds, chopped
- 4 tbsp shredded coconut
- 6-8 oz. crystallized ginger, chopped small
- 1/3 cup almond butter
- ¼ cup maple syrup
- 2 tablespoons plant or nut-based milk
- ½ cup Medjool dates, pitted and chopped
- 2 scoops vegan vanilla protein powder

**Directions:**

Mix together oats and cereal.

In saucepan over the medium low heat, mix maple syrup, almond butter, dates, milk and protein powder. Stirring constantly until melting.

Pour almond butter mixture over oats and cereal.

Transfer mixture into baking pan and press down.

Bake at 325 °F for 20 minutes.

# Fast & Chewy Gluten Free No-Bake Protein Bars

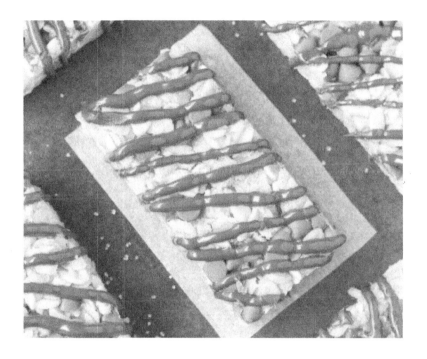

For added moisture, add ½ - 1 tsp of any variety milk.

**Makes:** 10 bars.

## Ingredients:

- 1 ¼ cups gluten-free rolled oats
- ½ cup vegan protein powder (we used unflavored)
- 1/3 cup + 1 tbsp rice crisp cereal
- ½ cup almond butter or sunflower seed butter
- ½ cup maple syrup
- 1 teaspoon pure vanilla extract
- 2 ½ -3 tablespoons mini dark chocolate chips
- ½ tablespoon coconut oil, melted

## Directions:

In a large bowl combine oats, protein powder, rice crisp, almond butter or sunflower seed butter, syrup, vanilla extract, Stirring well after each addition.

Press into 8x8 pan and freeze 30 minutes.

Meanwhile, melt chocolate chips and coconut oil together then drizzle over bars.

# 10 Almond Fudge No-Bake Bars

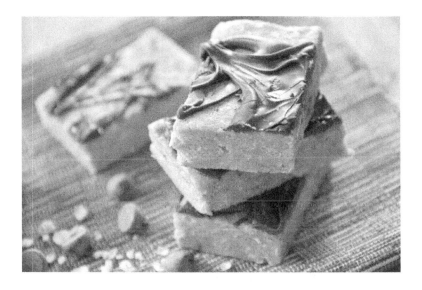

For extra deliciousness, melt chocolate and drizzle over these bars!

**Makes:** 8-10 bars.

## Ingredients:

- 1 cup oats, ground
- ½ cup quick oats
- 1/3 cup vanilla protein powder (I used whey)
- ½ cup crispy rice cereal
- ½ cup almond butter (or peanut butter)
- 1/3 cup honey
- 1 tsp. vanilla extract

## Directions:

Grind oats until a flour.

Mix together with oats, protein powder, crispy rice.

In small pot over medium heat, melt almond butter then stir in vanilla extract.

Pour melted butter and extract into dry ingredients then press down into 8x8 or 9x9 pan.

Refrigerate 30-45 minutes before slicing into bars.

# Brownie Protein Bars

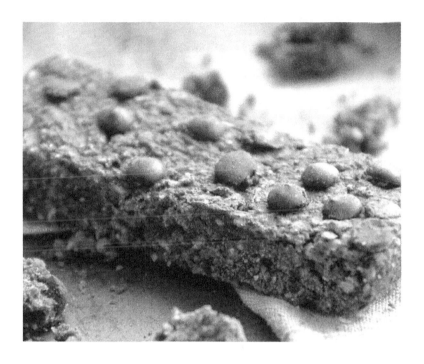

7.3 grams of protein.

**Makes:** 8-10 bars.

**Ingredients:**

- 1 cup black beans, washed and drained
- 2 ½ tbsp Dutch or regular cocoa powder
- ¼ cup + 3 tbsp chocolate protein powder
- Pinch of salt
- 1/3 cup maple syrup, agave, or organic honey
- ¼ tsp stevia
- 3 tbsp coconut or vegetable oil
- ½ tbsp vanilla extract
- ¼ tsp baking powder
- 2/3 cup chocolate chips

**Directions:**

Preheat oven to 350. Prepare 8x8 or 9x9 pan with non-stick cooking spray or parchment paper.

Combine in food processor black beans, cocoa powder, protein powder, salt, syrup, stevia, oil, extract, baking powder blending until smooth.

Bake bars 15 minutes, will firm upon sitting and cooling.

# Vegan Chocolate Peanut Butter Protein Bars

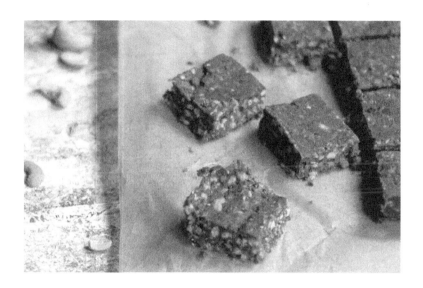

**Ingredients:**

- ¾ cup old-fashioned rolled oats
- ½ cup quick oats
- 1 scoop + 1 tbsp chocolate plant-based protein powder
- 1/3 cup + 2 tbsp organic brown rice crisp cereal
- ¼ cup maple syrup or agave
- 1/3 cup peanut butter
- 1 teaspoon vanilla extract
- 1-2 tablespoon carob or chocolate chips

**Directions:**

In a food processor combine rolled & quick oats, protein powder, brown rice cereal and blend.

In saucepan over medium heat melt together syrup or agave, peanut butter and extract.

Remove from heat, let cool, then pour over oat mixture.

Pour into pan and press evenly.

Melt carob or chocolate chips and drizzle over bars.

Cover and stick in refrigerator 30-45 minutes before slicing.

# 6-Step Easy Protein Bars

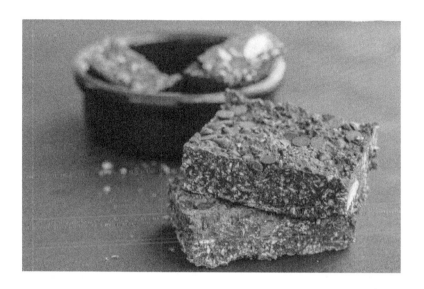

Make ahead! Keeps frozen for 1 month.

**Ingredients:**

- 1 cup almond butter, brought to room temp
- 2 ½ tablespoons almond milk
- 3 ½ tbsp brown rice syrup
- 1 tablespoon cocoa powder
- ½ cup protein powder
- ½ cup rolled oats

**Directions:**

Combine almond butter, almond milk, and syrup together and stir.

Add in cocoa powder, protein powder, rolled oats and stir.

Press into an 8x8 or 9x9 pan and chill in refrigerator 30-45 minutes.

# Easy Matcha Green Tea Protein Bars

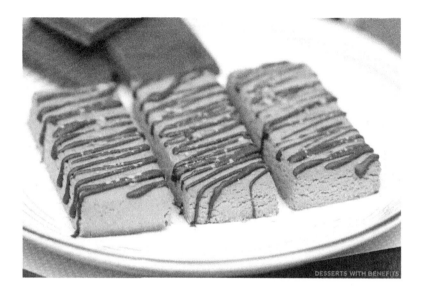

Melt and drizzle with white or dark chocolate!

**Makes:** 8-10 bars. 15 grams of protein.

**Ingredients:**

- 1/3 cup + 1 tbsp roasted almond butter
- ¾ cup + 2 tsp Unsweetened Vanilla Almond Milk
- 2/3 tsp Vanilla Crème-Flavored Stevia Extract
- 1/3 tsp Almond Extract
- ¾ cup + 1 tbsp lightly packed Vanilla Brown Rice Protein Powder
- ½ cup oat flour
- 1 ½ tbsp Matcha Powder

**Directions:**

In bowl mix together almond butter, almond milk, stevia, extract, protein powder, oat flour, Matcha powder.

Press dough into 8x8 pan and refrigerate overnight before slicing.

# Cranberry Protein Bars

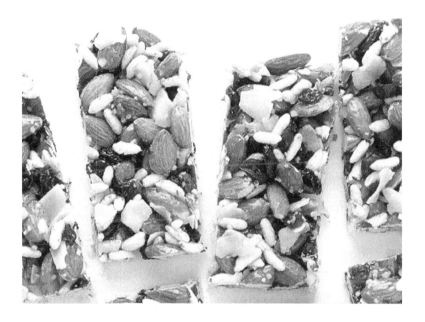

Beware, the wet ingredients will harden quickly once off heat!

**Makes:** 8-10 bars, 8g of protein.

## Ingredients:

- 2 cups almonds
- ½ - 2/3 cup puffed rice cereal
- ½ cup dried cranberries
- 1/3 cup coconut flakes
- ½ tablespoon hemp seeds
- 7 tbsp brown rice syrup
- 2 tablespoons honey, maple syrup, or agave
- 1 teaspoon vanilla extract

## Directions:

In a bowl stir together almonds, cereal, cranberries, hempseeds, and coconut. Set aside.

In saucepan over medium heat stir together syrup, honey and extract and let boil 4 ½ - 5 minutes.

Pour over dry mix, toss then press into 8x8 pan.

Cover and refrigerate 1 hour before slicing.

# Not Quite Brownies Protein Bars

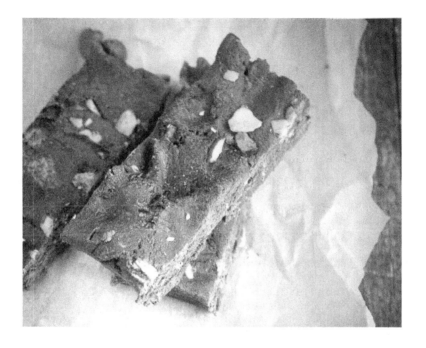

Try cookies and cream flavored powder!

**Makes:** 8-10 bars, 8 grams protein.

**Ingredients:**

- ¾ cup oat flour
- 3 ½ tbsp almond flour
- 2 tbsp vanilla whey protein powder
- 2 tbsp chocolate whey protein powder
- 2 ½ tablespoons dark cocoa powder
- 1 egg
- 1 tablespoon egg white
- 1/3 teaspoon stevia baking blend
- 3 tablespoons unsweetened applesauce
- 3 tablespoons plain Greek yogurt
- 3 tablespoons almond milk
- ¼ teaspoon of baking soda
- 2 – 3 tablespoons dark chocolate chips

**Directions:**

Preheat oven to 350 and prepare 8x8 pan with non-stick cooking spray and/or parchment paper.

In a separate bowl whisk together egg and stevia and set aside,

In a large bowl combine oat flour, almond flour, vanilla and chocolate protein powder, cocoa powder, baking soda. Stir well.

To that bowl stir in applesauce, egg white, yogurt, almond milk.

Pour in pan and bake 25-30 minutes.

Melt chocolate chips and drizzle over bars.

Cut into bars and keep store in refrigerator.

# Chocolate Raspberry Protein Squares

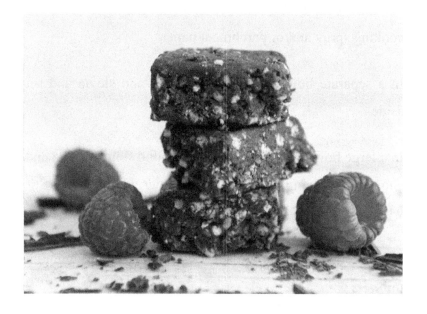

Made with all-natural sweeteners!

**Makes:** 8 – 10 bars, 11 g of protein.

**Ingredients:**

- ½ – 2/3 cup almond butter (peanut butter works too!)
- ¼ cup + 1 tbsp blue agave or honey
- ¾ - 1 cup instant rolled oats
- 4 tbsp chocolate protein powder
- 2-3 tbsp flaxseed
- ½ cup raspberries

**Directions:**

In a large bowl mix together oats, protein powder, and flaxseed; then, fold in raspberries.

In saucepan over medium-heat meld together almond butter with agave or honey until smooth.

Prepare a 5x9 loaf pan by placing parchment paper in it.

Pour in batter, even, let chill in refrigerator 45 minutes to 1 hour.

Store in air-tight container in refrigerator 5-7 days.

Try substituting blueberries for the raspberries!

# No-Bake Mint Protein Bars

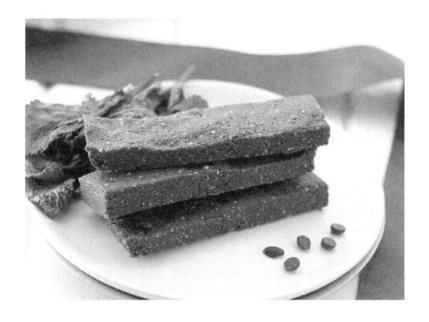

If you love Thin Mints, you'll love these.

**Makes:** 8-10 bars, 11.8 grams of protein.

## Ingredients:

- ¾ cup of dates, washed and pitted
- 1/3 cup cashew
- 1/3 cup of almonds
- ½ cup protein powder (if using whey protein add ½ tsp milk)
- 3 ½ tbsp cocoa powder
- ¼ tsp peppermint extract
- 1 ½ tbsp almond milk

## Directions:

In processor pulsate dates until pea sized.

Pulse in cashews, almonds until flour.

Add in protein powder, cocoa powder, extract, almond milk until dough forms a ball.

Place in 8x8 pan and refrigerate 30 minutes before slicing in bars.

# P.B. Dough Protein Dough

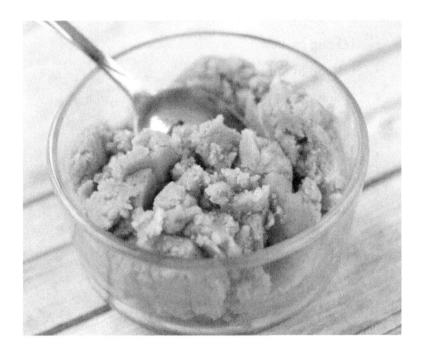

Great vegan option!

**Makes:** 8-10 bars, 8 grams of protein.

## Ingredients:

- ¼ cup rolled oats
- 10 large Medjool dates
- 1 cup raw cashews
- ½ cup protein powder
- 3 tablespoons peanut butter
- 2 tablespoons maple syrup

## Directions:

Blend oats to flour.

Top with protein powder, cashews, dates, peanut butter, syrup and blend until sticky (go past crumbly).

Pour into 8x8 dish, press down, and let chill in refrigerator 45 minutes – 1 hour.

Not sticky enough? Add ½ tsp more syrup. Need more p.b. flavor? Add another tbsp.

# Fudgy Red Velvet Protein Bars

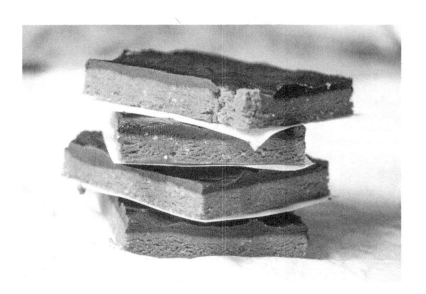

These delicious bars are all-natural!

**Makes:** 8-10 bars, 17 grams of protein per bar.

**Ingredients:**

- Between 1/3 – ½ cup beet juice
- ½ cup roasted almond butter
- ½ cup unsweetened vanilla almond milk
- 1 tbs natural butter
- 1½ tsp Vanilla Crème-Flavored Stevia Extract
- 1¼ cups Chocolate Brown Rice Protein Powder (stay away from whey or egg protein)
- 1/3 cup Oat Flour
- 2-3 tbsp chocolate chips or carob chips, melted
- 1 tbsp coconut oil, melted

## Directions:

Preheat oven to 350, wash beets, wrap in foil then roast on baking sheet 1 ½ hours.

Remove foil and skin then puree.

Blend together beet juice, almond butter, milk, butter, extract, protein powder, oat flour until thick like cookie dough.

Pour into 8x8 or 9x9 pan, cover, and refrigerate 5 hours to overnight before slicing.

Melt chips and coconut oil together stirring well then drizzle over bars.

# Apple Pie Protein Bars

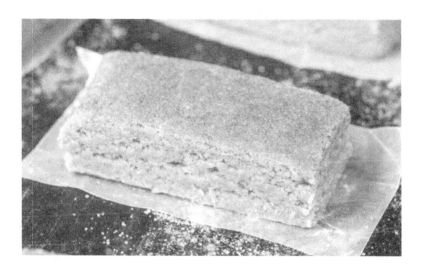

A taste of dessert without the fat and sugar!

**Makes:** 8-10 bars, 10 g of protein.

**Ingredients:**

- 1 2/3 -2 cups of gluten free oat flour -or- 1 cup coconut flour
- 10-12 scoops vanilla vegan or you can use paleo friendly protein powder
- ¼ tsp cinnamon
- ½ tsp stevia or natural granulated sweetener
- 1/5 tsp nutmeg
- 1 /2 tsp apple pie spice
- ½ cup brown rice syrup (or maple syrup for paleo)
- ¼ cup of almond butter (or any nut butter)
- ¾ dairy free milk
- ½ cup coconut flour
- ½ cup of unsweetened applesauce

**Directions:**

Combine flours, protein, sweetener, cinnamon, apple pie spice, nutmeg and stir well.

Melt together nut butter and syrup then pour into dry ingredients and add applesauce.

Slowly beat milk in.

Pour into 8x8 or 9x9 pan and refrigerate 1 hour before slicing.

# No Bake Cinnamon Roll Protein Bars

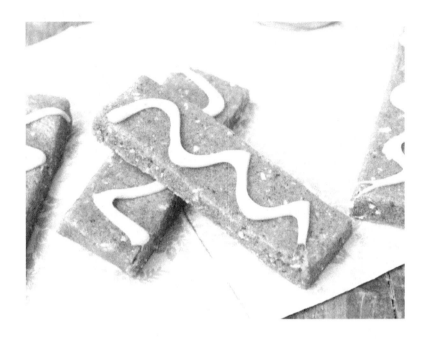

Stabilize your B.P. with these cinnamon bars!

**Makes:** 8-10 bars, 9 g of protein.

**Ingredients:**

- 1 cup raw, cashews
- ¾ cup, pitted dates
- ½ cup + 3 tbsp vanilla protein powder
- 1/3 tsp cinnamon
- Pinch of sea salt
- ¼ + 2 tbsp cup rolled oats
- 1 tbsp almond milk (or milk alternative)
- For the protein drizzle:
- 1 scoop (2 tbsp) vanilla protein powder
- 2/3 tbsp almond milk (or other non-dairy milk), if more is needed add ¼ tsp at a time

## Directions:

Process cashews and dates 2-4 minutes.

Add in protein powder, oats, cinnamon, salt and blend until dough forms a ball.

Stir in milk.

Pour dough into 8x8 or 9x9 pan and let chill in refrigerator 30 minutes.

Mix together vanilla protein powder and milk then place in piping bag.

Draw desired patterns on bars with mix then freeze 20 minutes.

# Banana No Bake Protein Bars

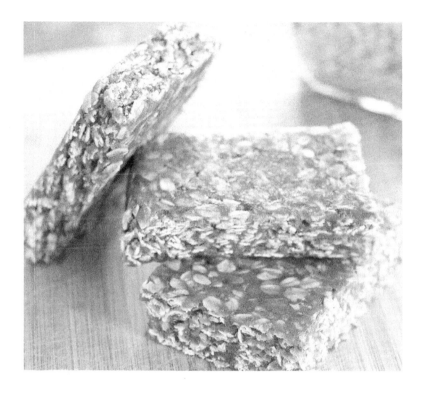

Use 1 jar of baby banana puree for the banana mash!

**Makes:** 8-10 bars, 8g of protein.

**Ingredients:**

- 2 cups of gluten free oat flour -or-1 cup coconut flour
- ½ cup of vanilla vegan or you can use paleo friendly protein powder
- ½ cup coconut flour -or- oat flour
- 2/3 tbsp cinnamon
- 1 tbsp granulated sweetener of choice
- ½ cup brown rice syrup (sub maple syrup in the paleo version)
- 3 tbsp almond butter (can sub any nut butter)
- ¼ cup chopped nuts of choice (optional)
- 1 small banana, mashed
- ½ tbsp dairy free milk +more as need 1/3 tsp at a time

**Directions:**

Combine flours, protein powder, granulated sweetener, cinnamon. Mix well and set aside.

Melt together nut butter and rice syrup then add to dry ingredients along with banana mash and nuts.

Slowly stir in milk.

Pour into 8x8 or 9x9 dish and let chill in refrigerator 1 hour before slicing.

# Mocha Protein Squares

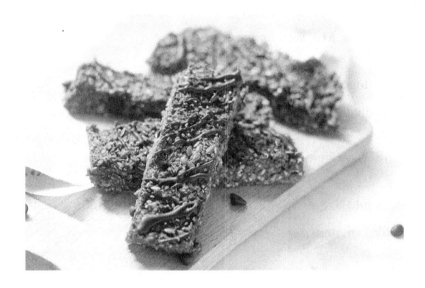

Tweak the amounts of sweetener and espresso to your tastes!

**Makes:** 8-10 bars, 8 grams of protein.

## Ingredients:

- ½ cup unflavored whey protein isolate
- 3 ½ tbsp coconut flour
- 3 1/3 tbsp almond flour
- 3 teaspoons unsweetened cacao powder
- 1 tbsp coconut sugar
- ½ cup -or- 4 oz espresso, freshly brewed and cooled
- 2-3 tbsp dark chocolate
- 1 tbsp coconut oil (optional)

## Directions:

In a large bowl combine whey protein, flours, cacao powder, coconut sugar.

Stir in espresso (don't worry if mixture still seems kind of dry or crumbly)

Cover and refrigerate 1 hour.

Melt chocolate and coconut oil together then drizzle over bars. Keep refrigerated

# P.B. Chip Protein Squares

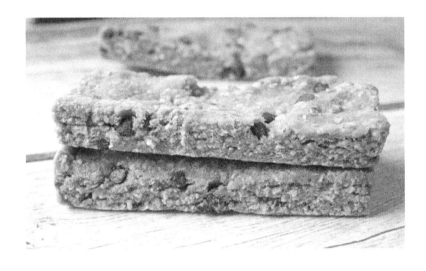

Add in white chocolate just for something different!

**Makes:** 8 -10 bars, 16 grams of protein.

**Ingredients:**

- ¾ tbsp maple syrup
- ¾ tsp vanilla extract
- 1/3 cup low-fat cottage cheese
- 1/3 tsp cinnamon
- ¼ cup unsweetened almond milk
- 6-7 pitted Medjool dates
- Pinch of sea salt
- ¾ cup organic peanut butter
- 4 ½ - 5 scoops vanilla protein powder -or- egg white protein powder
- 1/3 cup oat flour
- 3 cup mini chocolate chips I used Enjoy Life brand
- 3 tbsp slivered almonds
- 2-3 tbsp mini dark chocolate chips
- 1 tbsp coconut oil

**Directions:**

Blend together maple syrup, extract, cottage cream, cinnamon, almond milk and salt until smooth.

Along with nut butter, transfer to a large bowl, blend, then stir in flours.

Pour evenly into an 8x8 or 9x9 pan and refrigerate 2 hours.

Melt together chocolate chips and coconut oil and drizzle on top of bars. Or slice bars and dip into chocolate.

# Sweet Potato Protein Squares

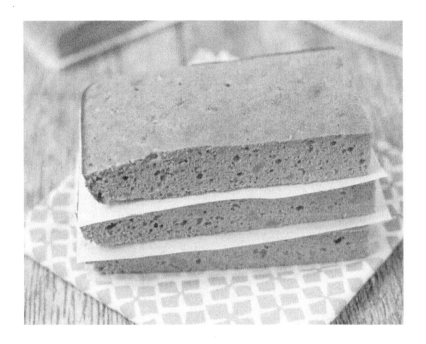

Add a dash of nutmeg too!

**Makes:** 8- 10 bars, 13 grams of protein.

## Ingredients:

- 1 cup mashed sweet potato
- ¾ tsp vanilla
- ¾ tsp + a pinch of cinnamon
- 1 tbsp maple syrup
- 2 eggs
- ¼ cup + 1 tbsp nut butter
- 1/3 cup plain yogurt
- 1 tbsp coconut oil
- ¼ tsp baking powder
- ½ cup vanilla or chocolate protein powder
- 2-3 tbsp mini chocolate chips

## Directions:

Blend together sweet potato mash, vanilla, cinnamon, maple syrup, eggs, nut butter and yogurt.

Add in baking powder and protein powder and mix until well combined.

Pour into 8x8 pan and bake 11-13 minutes.

Let cool and meanwhile, melt together chocolate chips and coconut oil then drizzle over cooled bars.

# Lemon Protein Bars

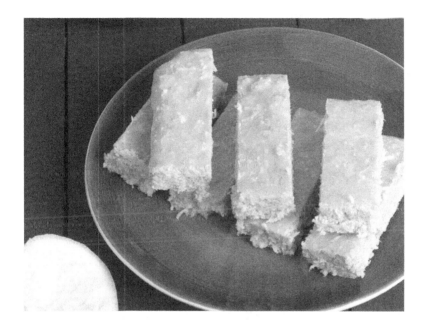

Blueberries and strawberries make nice flavors too!

**Makes:** 8 – 10 bars, 11 grams of protein.

## Ingredients:

- ¾ cup protein powder
- ½ cup almond meal
- 1/3 cup coconut flour
- ½ cup shredded coconut
- 3 large eggs, liquid eggs, vegan eggs, etc.
- 3 tbsp maple syrup
- ¼ cup + 1 tbsp lemon juice
- 1 tbsp chia seeds
- ¼ cup coconut milk
- Optional Drizzle
- 2-3 tbsp mini dark chocolate chips
- 1 tbsp coconut oil

**Directions:**

Preheat oven to 350.

Blend together protein powder, almond flour, coconut flour, shredded coconut, eggs, syrup, lemon juice, chia seeds.

Slowly stream in milk.

Pour mixture into 8x8 or 9x9 pan and let chill 30 minutes 1 hour in refrigerator.

Let bars cool and melt together chips and coconut oil then drizzle over bars. Or, cut into bars and dip into chocolate.

# Vegan Joy Protein Bars

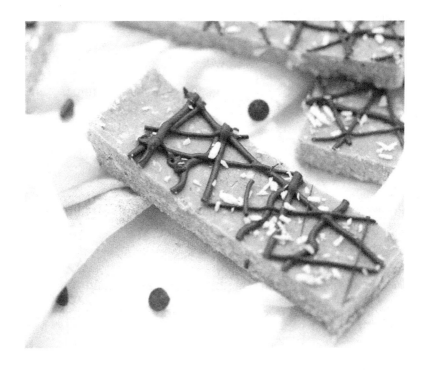

If you like Almond Joy bars, you'll love these.

**Makes:** 8-10 bars, 8 grams of protein.

**Ingredients:**

- 1 cups oat flour
- 1 ½ tbsp coconut flour
- ½ cup coconut flakes
- ½ cup vegan protein powder
- 1 ½ tbsp coconut oil
- ½ tsp almond extract
- 3 ½ tbsp maple syrup
- 3 ½ tbsp coconut milk add ½ tsp, as needed
- 2-3 tbsp dairy-free chocolate chips, melted
- 2 tsp coconut oil

**Directions:**

In a large bowl combine coconut flour, oat flour protein powder and coconut flakes.

In separate bowl combine coconut oil, vanilla, maple syrup, coconut milk.

Pour wet ingredients into dry ingredients and stir.

Pour into 8x8 or 9x9 dish and let chill in refrigerator 30 minutes.

Melt together chocolate chips and coconut oil then drizzle over bars.

# Easy Protein Bar

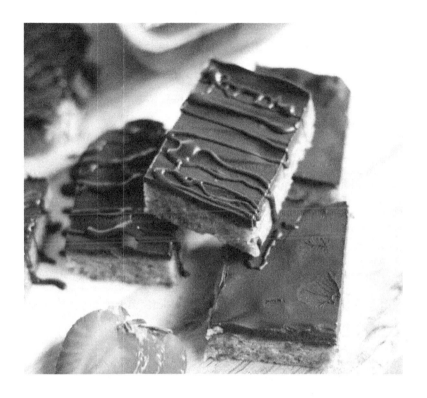

2 pot bars!

**Makes:** 8 – 10, 7 grams of protein.

**Ingredients:**

- ½ cup whole milk
- ¾ cup natural chunky peanut butter
- 2–3 tbsp honey, agave, or maple syrup
- 2 scoops chocolate or vanilla whey protein powder
- 1 2/3 cups old fashioned rolled oats
- 2-3 tbsp mini dark chocolate chips for drizzling
- 1 tbsp coconut oil

**Directions:**

In saucepan over medium-high heat combine milk, peanut butter, sweetener, whey protein powder, and mix until well combined.

Remove from heat and stir in oats.

Let chill in refrigerator 30 minutes before slicing.

Melt chocolate chips and coconut oil together then drizzle onto bars or dip them into mix.

# No Chocolate Peanut Butter Protein Bars

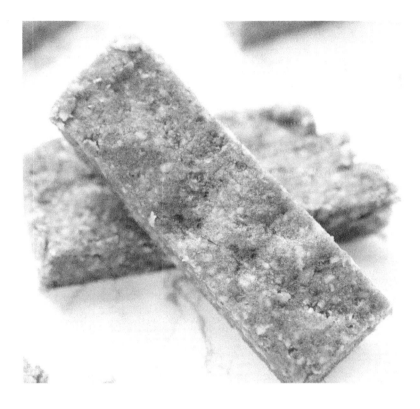

Sub French vanilla protein powder for vanilla.

**Makes:** 8 – 10 bars, 13 grams of protein.

## Ingredients:

- 1 2/3 cups rolled oats
- 6-8 Medjool dates, washed & pitted
- 2/3 cup peanut butter, room temp.
- ¼ cup + 1 tbsp honey
- ½ teaspoon vanilla extract
- 2-3 scoops vanilla protein powder

## Directions:

Blend oats into oat flour.

Add in dates, peanut butter, honey, vanilla extract, protein powder.

Pour into 8x8 or 9x9 dish and let chill 30 minutes in refrigerator.

# Turmeric Crispy Rice Protein Snack

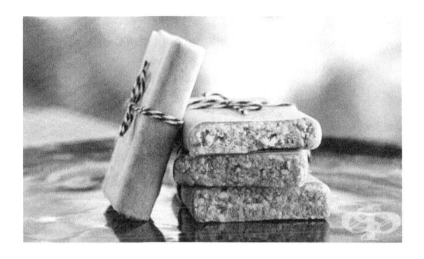

Sub ginger for the turmeric!

**Makes:** 8 – 10 bars, 11 grams of protein.

## Ingredients:

- 3 ½ cups crispy rice cereal
- ¾ cup smooth or chunky peanut butter
- 1 cup chocolate chips
- 1 tbsp honey
- 1 tsp turmeric
- 3 cup marshmallows
- 2/3 cup honey roasted peanuts -or- chopped walnuts

## Directions:

In a large pot melt together peanut butter, chocolate, honey, turmeric, and marshmallows.

Remove from heat and stir add cereal and honey roasted peanuts.

# Gingerbread Spice Protein Bars

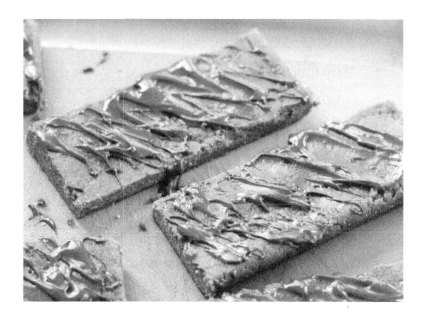

Although not gluten free, for more gingerbread flavor sub molasses for honey!

**Makes:** 8- 10 bars, 13 grams of protein.

**Ingredients:**

- ½ cup brown rice protein powder
- 2 ½ tbsp coconut flour
- ¾ tsp ground ginger
- ½ tsp cinnamon
- ¼ tsp nutmeg
- 1/6 tsp cloves
- 1/3 cup + 2 tbsp natural nut butter
- 1 ½ tbsp coconut oil
- ½ tbsp honey, maple syrup, or agave
- ¼ cup dairy milk (to add more stir in 1/3 tsp at a time)

**Directions:**

In a large bowl combine protein powder, coconut flour, ginger, cinnamon, nutmeg.

Melt together nut butter, coconut oil, and sweetener together.

Mix together wet and dry mixes.

Slowly stir in milk.

Pour into 8x8 or 9x9 pan and chill in refrigerator 30 minutes.

# Paleo Almond Mango Coconut Protein

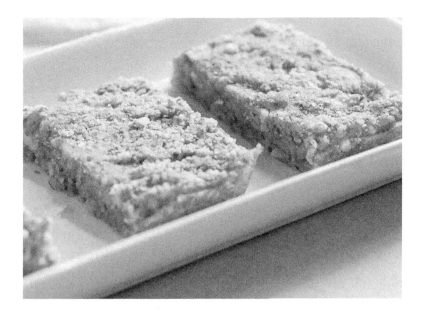

Try dried pomegranates!

**Makes:** 8 – 10 bars, 9 grams of protein.

**Ingredients:**

- 3 cups almonds
- 4 tbsp dried Mango
- 2/3 cup coconut flakes
- ½ cup egg white powder or ¼ cup protein powder
- ¼ cup + 1 tbsp honey or maple syrup
- ½ tsp vanilla extract
- 2/3 tsp cinnamon
- 1/3 cup hot water

**Directions:**

Mix together hot water and honey or maple syrup.

Grind mango 1-2 minutes then add almonds, coconut flakes, protein powder, cinnamon.

Combine wet and dry mixtures then press into 8x8 or 9x9 pan.

Let chill in refrigerator 30 minutes before slicing.

# Vanilla Hempseed Protein Bars

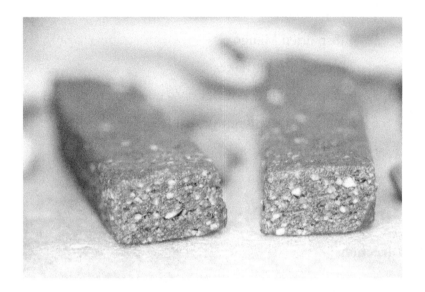

Try various nuts and seeds!

**Makes:** 8 – 10 bars, 9 grams of protein.

**Ingredients:**

- 2/3 cup vanilla protein
- 3 ½ tbsp almond flour
- 1 ½ tbsp coconut flour
- 1 tbsp cacao powder
- 1/3 tsp cinnamon
- 1/3 tsp cardamom
- Pinch of ginger
- Pinch of nutmeg
- Pinch of cloves
- ½ cup sunflower butter (or a natural nut butter)
- 2 tbsp honey or brown rice syrup
- ½ tbsp coconut oil, melted
- 2 ½ tbsp non-dairy milk
- 2-3 tbsp mini chocolate chips
- 2/3 tsp coconut oil
- 1-2 tbsp hemp seeds

**Directions:**

In a large bowl combine protein powder, almond flour, coconut flour, cacao powder, cinnamon, cardamom, ginger, nutmeg, cloves, mix well and set aside.

In another bowl mix together sunflower butter, honey, melted coconut oil.

Mix the wet and dry ingredients and slowly stir in milk.

Press into 8x8 or 9x9 dish and chill in refrigerator 30 minutes.

Melt together chocolate chips and coconut oil then stir in hemp seeds.

Drizzle over bars.

# Chewy Protein Squares

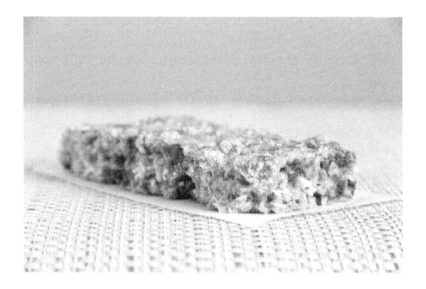

Great for adding in seeds or dried fruit.

**Makes:** 8 – 10 bars, 9 grams of protein.

**Ingredients:**

- 1 tsp. vanilla extract
- ½ cup chocolate or vanilla protein powder
- ¼ cup unsweetened cocoa powder
- 1 ¾ cups quick oats
- ½ cup mini chocolate chips

**Directions:**

Preheat oven to 350 and prepare 8x8 or 9x9 dish.

Blend together almond butter, dates, almond milk, and vanilla.

Add protein powder, cocoa.

By hand stir in oats and chocolate chips until just covered then pour into prepared dish and bake

15-20 minutes.

# Almond, Honey, and Flax Protein Bars

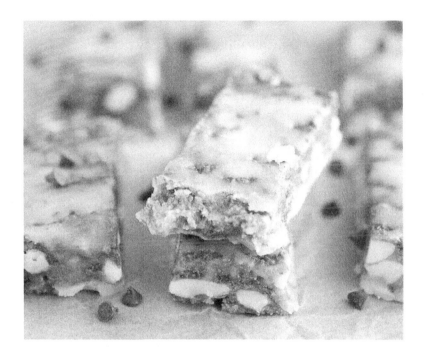

Any nut butter will work.

**Makes:** 8 – 10 bars, 9 grams of protein.

## Ingredients:

- ½ cup of oat flour
- ¼ cup + ½ tbsp vanilla protein powder
- 3 tbsp maple syrup
- 1 cup of honey
- 1 ½ - 2 tbsp flax
- 1 cup almond butter
- 2 Tablespoons of Almond Milk

## Directions:

Combine almond milk, almond butter, maple syrup and mix well.

In a separate bowl combine oat flour and protein powder.

Combine wet and dry mixtures.

Press into 8x8 or 9x9 dish and let chill 45 minutes in refrigerator.

# Salted Caramel Protein Bars

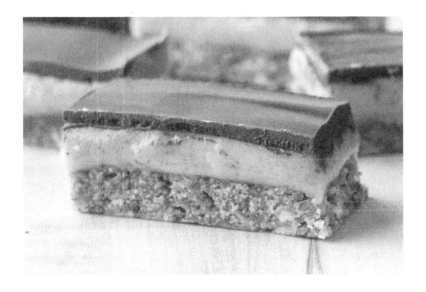

Use your favorite flavor of whey protein!

**Makes:** 8 – 10 bars, 10 grams of protein.

**Ingredients:**

- ¼ cup salted pretzel caramel peanut butter
- ¼ cup coconut oil, melted
- 1/3 cup milk
- 3 ½ tbsp whey protein powder
- 1/3 cup coconut flour
- 3 tbsp brownie coconutter (such as Sweet Spreads)
- 1/3 cup pretzels, crushed

**Directions:**

Whisk together peanut butter, coconut oil, milk.

In another bowl whisk together protein powder, coconut flour.

Combine wet and dry ingredients.

Press dough into 8x8 or 9x9 pan and chill 1 hour.

Melt coconutter and spread on bars topping with crushed pretzels.

# Coconut Pomegranate Protein Bars

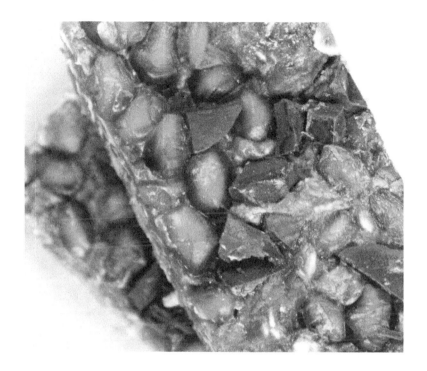

Substitute dried cranberries for the dried pomegranate!

**Makes:** 8 – 10 bars, 10 grams of protein.

**Ingredients:**

- 3 heaping tbsp coconut flakes
- ¼ cup dried pomegranates
- ¼ cup almond butter
- 3 tbsp almond flour
- 1 tbsp flax meal
- 2 ½ tbsp coconut oil
- 1 tbsp raw honey or agave
- 2 eggs or ¼ cup liquid egg substitute
- 6 scoops coconut protein powder
- 2-3 tbsp dark chocolate chunks
- 1 tbsp coconut oil

**Directions:**

Preheat oven to 350 and prepare 8x8 or 9x9 dish.

Mix together coconut flakes, dried pomegranates, almond butter, almond flour, flax meal, coconut oil, honey/agave, egg or substitute, coconut protein powder.

Press into pan and bake 30 minutes.

If desired, melt chocolate and coconut oil together then drizzle on top of bars.

# Chai Spice Protein Bars

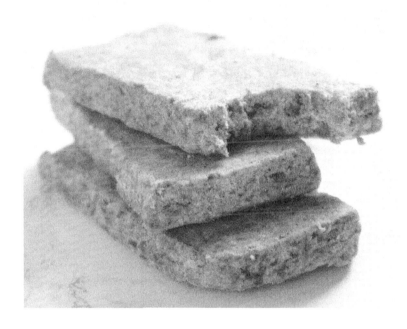

Great for breakfast!

**Makes:** 8 – 10 bars, 11 grams of protein.

**Ingredients:**

- 1 cups whole wheat or gluten free flour
- 1 ½ scoop protein powder
- 1 tbsp coconut sugar
- ½ tsp vanilla extract
- ½ tsp cinnamon
- ¼ tsp cardamom
- ¼ tsp ginger
- ¼ tsp cloves
- ½ tsp baking soda
- ¼ tsp all spice
- 2 eggs or 2 tbsp egg substitute
- 1/3 cup + 1 tbsp maple syrup
- 1 tbsp coconut oil, melted

**Directions:**

Preheat oven to 350 and prepare 8x8 or 9x9 dish.

In a large bowl combine wheat or g.f. flour, protein powder, sugar, baking soda, cinnamon, cardamom, ginger, cloves, and allspice.

In another whisk together eggs or substitute, syrup, coconut oil, vanilla.

Combine wet and dry ingredients then pour into pan.

Bale 15-20 minutes

# Coconut Matcha Protein Squares

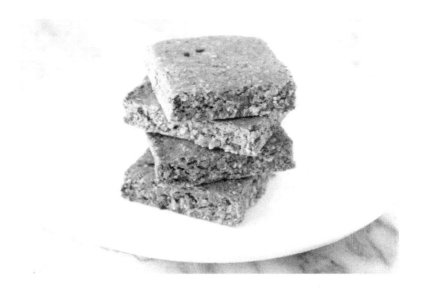

Vegan and gluten free!

**Makes:** 8 – 10 bars, 13 grams of protein

**Ingredients:**

- 1 cup coarsely chopped dates washed & pitted
- 1/3 cup cashews
- 1/3 cup almonds
- ¾ tsp of vanilla bean or you can use pure vanilla extract
- 1/5 cup hemp seeds
- 2-3 tbsp cacao nibs
- 1 tbsp Matcha powder
- 2-3 tbsp coconut flakes

**Directions:**

Blend together dates, almonds, cashews, hemp seeds, vanilla, and ½ Matcha powder.

Add nibs in short 4-5 second pulses to disperse throughout mixture.

Press mixture into 8x8 or 9x9 pan, top with coconut flakes and remaining Matcha powder, and refrigerate 30 minutes.

# Quick Strawberry Protein Bars

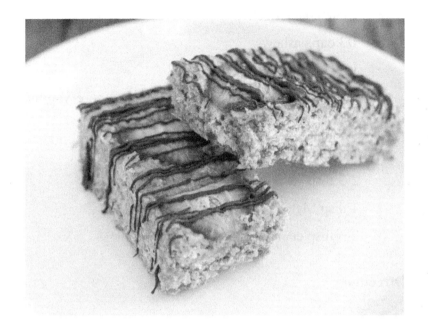

Quick, easy, and to the point!

**Makes:** 8 -10 bars, 10 grams of protein.

## Ingredients:

- 2/3 cup all-natural nut butter
- 2/3 cup oat flour
- ½ cup honey
- 2 ½ scoops of strawberry flavored protein powder

## Directions:

Mix together nut butter, oat flour, honey, protein powder.

Press into 8x8 or 9x9 dish and refrigerate 1 hour before slicing.

# Quinoa Protein Bars

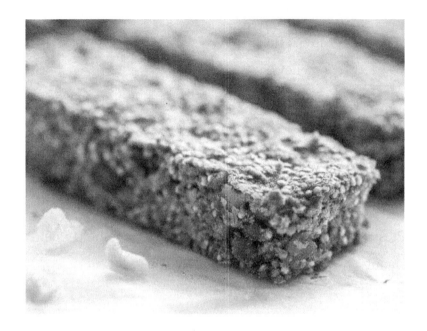

Try cashews instead of almonds.

**Makes:** 8 – 10 bars, 7 grams of protein.

**Ingredients:**

- 1/3 cup + 1 tbsp dry quinoa
- 1/3 cup raw almonds; chopped coarsely
- ½ cup chia seeds
- 1/3 tsp. pink Himalayan salt
- ¾ cup rolled oats gluten free
- 2/3 tsp cardamom
- 2/3 tsp cinnamon
- 1/3 cup honey
- 1 ½ tbsp. ground flax seeds
- 1/3 cup almond butter
- ¼ cup brown rice syrup

**Directions:**

Preheat oven 350 then prepare an 8x8 or 9x9 dish.

In large bowl combine chia seeds, quinoa, flaxseeds, rolled oats, salt, cinnamon, raw almonds and cardamom.

In microwave safe dish cook for 1-minute almond butter, brown rice syrup, and honey.

Combine wet and dry ingredients.

Press into prepared dish and cook 15-20 minutes.

# Sea Salt & Chocolate Protein Squares

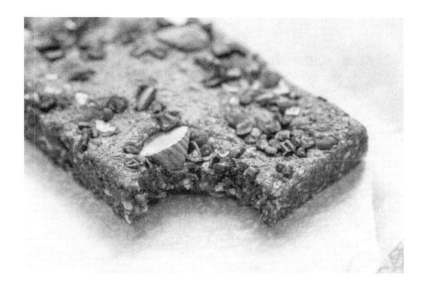

Try strawberry powder instead of cocoa.

**Makes:** 8-10 bars, 8 grams of protein.

**Ingredients:**

- ¾ cup whole almonds
- ¾ cup raw cashews
- 2/3 cup pitted dates
- ½ cup egg white protein powder
- 2 tablespoons cocoa powder
- 2 tablespoons water
- 2-3 tbsp cacao nibs, for topping (optional)

**Directions:**

Blend together almonds and cashews 4 minutes.

Add dates, egg white powder, cocoa powder, 2 tbsp water until dough is crumbly.

Press into 8x8 or 9x9 pan and, if desired, press leftover almonds, cacao nibs, and/or salt into bars for topping.

Cover and refrigerate 45 minutes – 1 hour before slicing.

# Cherry Almond Protein Bars

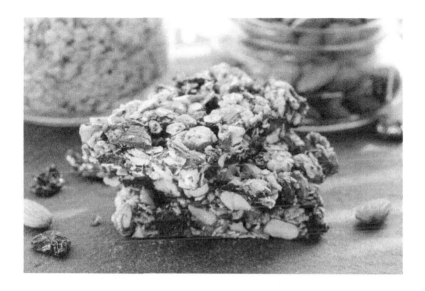

Great for adding in plant-based proteins and seeds!

**Makes:** 8 - 10 bars, 9 grams of protein.

**Ingredients:**

- 2 cups old fashioned rolled oats
- ½ cup slivered almonds
- 1/3 cup unsweetened shredded coconut
- ¼ cup honey
- 3 tbsp butter, cut into cubes
- 3 ½ tbsp light brown sugar, packed
- 1/6 tsp almond extract
- 2-3 tbsp cacao nibs
- 1/3 cup dried tart cherries, coarsely chopped
- 2.5 ounces bittersweet chocolate

**Directions:**

Preheat oven to 350 and prepare a baking sheet and an 8x8 or 9x9 dish.

Combine oats, almonds and coconut and spread out on baking sheet.

Bake 4 minutes, flip, bake 4 more. Let cool and transfer to bowl.

In saucepan over medium heat bring to a boil and stir together honey, butter, brown sugar until all is dissolved.

Remove, stir in extract and pour over oat mixture.

Stir in nibs and cherries.

Press into 8x8 or 9x9 pan and refrigerate 1-2 hours before cutting.

# Cherry Almond Vanilla Protein Bars

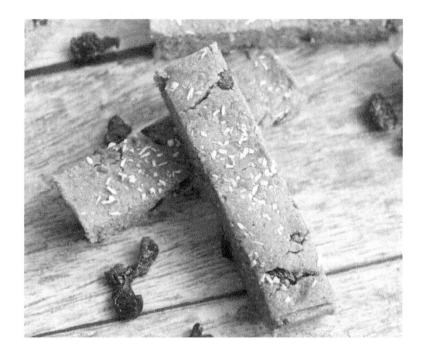

Try chocolate protein powder!

**Makes:** 8 – 10 bars, 13 grams of protein.

**Ingredients:**

- 2 cups of old fashioned rolled oats
- 3 scoops vanilla protein powder
- 1/3 cup shredded coconut
- ½ cup slivered almonds
- ¼ cup honey
- 3 tbsp butter, cut into cubes
- 3 ½ tbsp light brown sugar, packed
- 1/6 teaspoon almond extract
- 2-3 tbsp cacao nibs
- ½ cup dried tart cherries, coarsely chopped
- 2.5 ounces bittersweet chocolate

## Directions:

Preheat oven to 350 and prepare a baking sheet and an 8x8 or 9x9 dish.

Combine oats, almonds and coconut and spread out on baking sheet.

Bake 4 minutes, flip, bake 4 more. Let cool, transfer to bowl stir in protein powder.

In saucepan over medium heat bring to a boil and stir together honey, butter, brown sugar until all is dissolved.

Remove, stir in extract and pour over oat mixture.

Stir in nibs and cherries.

Press into 8x8 or 9x9 pan and refrigerate 1-2 hours before cutting.

# French Vanilla Mint Protein Bars

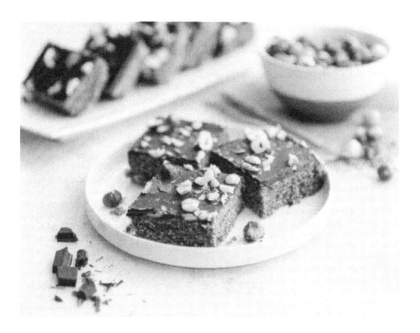

If using vanilla protein powder add ¼ tsp vanilla extract.

**Makes:** 8 – 10 bars, 11 grams of protein.

## Ingredients:

- ¾ cup of dates
- ½ cup cashews
- ½ cup of almonds
- ¾ cup French vanilla protein powder
- 3 tbsp cocoa powder
- ¼ tsp peppermint extract
- 2 tbsp almond milk (2 ½ - 3 tbsp if using whey protein powder)
- ¼ tsp sea salt

## Directions:

Blend dates, cashews and almonds until finely ground.

Add in protein powder, cocoa powder, peppermint extract, almond milk, and salt until ball is formed.

Press into an 8x8 or 9x9 dish, cover, and refrigerate 20-30 minutes before slicing.

# Cinnamon Banana Protein Bars

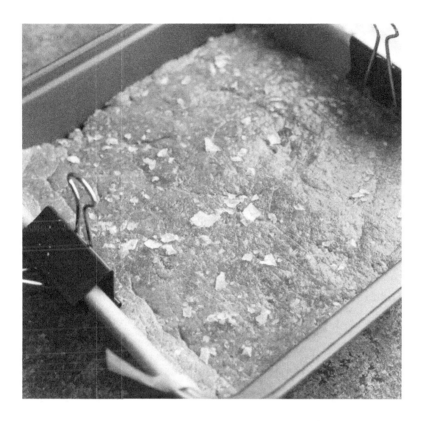

Sunflower seeds or soy seeds are also great additions!

**Makes:** 8 – 10 bars, 7 grams of protein.

## Ingredients:

- 1 cup mashed banana
- ¾ can chickpeas
- ½ cup + 1 tbsp almond butter -or- peanut butter
- 1/3 cup ground flaxseed -or- hempseed
- 2/3 Tbsp cinnamon
- ¼ tsp nutmeg

## Directions:

Preheat oven to 350 and prepare 8x8 or 9x9 dish.

Blend together mashed banana, chickpeas, nut butter flax or hemp seed, cinnamon, nutmeg.

Pres into pan and bake 18-25 minutes.

# Cranberry Banana Protein Bars

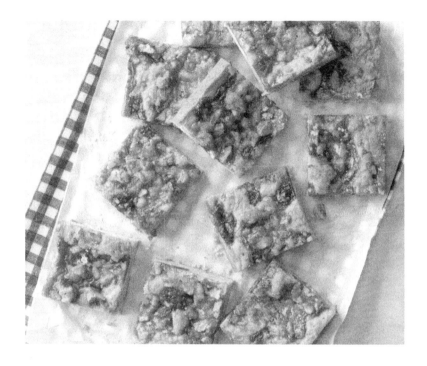

Try raisins or dried pineapple!

**Makes:** 8 – 10 bars, 7 grams of protein.

## Ingredients:

- 1 cup mashed banana
- ¾ can chickpeas
- ½ cup + 1 tbsp almond butter -or- peanut butter
- ½ - 2/3 cup dried cranberries
- 1/3 tsp cloves (optional)
- ¼ tsp nutmeg (optional)

## Directions:

Preheat oven to 350 and prepare 8x8 or 9x9 dish.

Blend together mashed banana, chickpeas, nut butter, cranberries, cloves, nutmeg.

Press into pan and bake 18-25 minutes.

# Chocolate Banana Mint Protein Bars

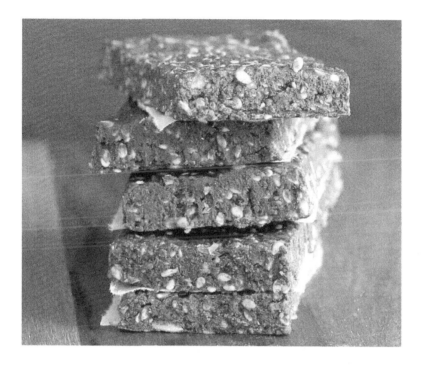

Try raisins or dried pineapple!

**Makes:** 8 – 10 bars, 7 grams of protein.

**Ingredients:**

- 2/3 cup mashed banana
- 1/3 can chickpeas
- ½ cup almond butter -or- peanut butter
- ½ cup dark chocolate chips
- 1/3 tsp peppermint extract

**Directions:**

Preheat oven to 350 and prepare 8x8 or 9x9 dish.

Blend together mashed banana, chickpeas, nut butter, chocolate chips and extract.

Press into pan and bake 18-25 minutes.

# Black Brownie Fudge Protein Squares

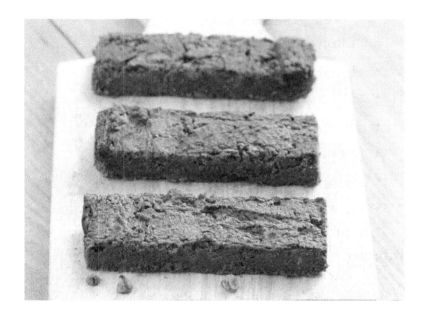

Also, Makes a great dessert!

**Makes:** 8 -10 bars, 8 grams of protein.

**Ingredients:**

- 1 cup black beans drained and rinsed
- 1 tbsp chocolate protein powder
- 1 tbsp peanut butter protein powder
- 3 tbsp cocoa powder
- 3 tbsp coconut oil
- 1 tbsp turbinado sugar
- ½ teaspoon vanilla extract
- ½ cup mini semi-sweet chocolate chips

**Directions:**

Preheat oven to 350 and prepare 8x8 or 9x9 dish.

Blend together black beans, both protein powders, cocoa powder, coconut oil, sugar, extract so dough is somewhat firm.

Press into pan and cook 15-30 minutes.

Let cool 30 minutes to 1 hour before slicing.

# Author's Afterthoughts

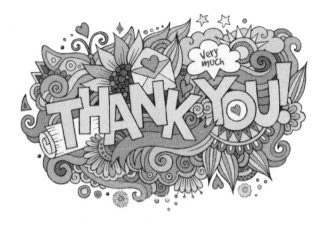

**Thanks ever so much to each of my cherished readers for investing the time to read this book!**

I know you could have picked from many other books, but you chose this one. So, a big thanks for reading all the way to the end. If you enjoyed this book or received value from it, I'd like to ask you for a favor. Please take a few minutes to **post an honest and heartfelt review on** *Amazon.com.* Your support does make a difference and helps to benefit other people.

*Thanks!*

**Julia Chiles**

# About the Author

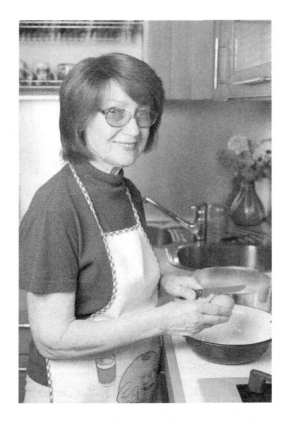

**Julia Chiles**

(1951-present)

Julia received her culinary degree from Le Counte' School of Culinary Delights in Paris, France. She enjoyed cooking more than any of her former positions. She lived in Montgomery, Alabama most of her life. She married Roger

Chiles and moved with him to Paris as he pursued his career in journalism. During the time she was there, she joined several cooking groups to learn the French cuisine, which inspired her to attend school and become a great chef.

Julia has achieved many awards in the field of food preparation. She has taught at several different culinary schools. She is in high demand on the talk show circulation, sharing her knowledge and recipes. Julia's favorite pastime is learning new ways to cook old dishes.

Julia is now writing cookbooks to add to her long list of achievements. The present one consists of favorite recipes as well as a few culinary delights from other cultures. She expands everyone's expectations on how to achieve wonderful dishes and not spend a lot of money. Julia firmly believes a wonderful dish can be prepare out of common household staples.

If anyone is interested in collecting Julia's cookbooks, check out your local bookstores and online. They are a big seller whatever venue you choose to purchase from.

Made in the USA
Las Vegas, NV
13 August 2025

26292085R10080